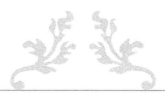

AN HEALTHY AIR FRYER COOKBOOK

Over 50 Affordable, Quick And Budget Friendly Recipes

Laura Clark

this book has been derived from various sources. Please consult a licensed professional before attempting any techniques outlined in this book.

By reading this document, the reader agrees that under no circumstances is the author responsible for any losses, direct or indirect, which are incurred as a result of the use of information contained within this document, including, but not limited to, errors, omissions, or inaccuracies.

Table of Contents

INTRODUCTION 9

BREAKFAST RECIPES 12

1. Spicy Hash Brown Potatoes 12

2. Sage and Pear Sausage Patties 14

3. Bacon Bombs 15

4. Morning Potatoes 16

5. Breakfast Pockets 17

6. Avocado Flautas 18

7. Cheese Sandwiches 20

8. Sausage Cheese Wraps 22

9. Sausage Burritos 23

10. Sausage Patties 24

11. Spicy Sweet Potato Hash 25

LUNCH RECIPES 27

12. Olives and Zucchini Cakes 27

13. Fluffy Strawberry Muffins 28

14. Paleo Blueberry Muffins 30

15. Orange Cardamom Muffins with Coconut Butter Glaze 32

16. Bacon and Egg Cups 34

17. Breadsticks 35

18. Butter Crackers 37

19. Homemade Almond Crackers 39

20. Pepperoni Chips 41

21. 3-Ingredient Flourless Cheesy Breadsticks 42

22. Cauliflower Breadsticks 44

23. Breadsticks with Mozzarella Dough 46

24. Bacon Onion Cookies 48

25. Cinnamon Swirl Cookies... 50

26. Peanut Butter Cookies 52

27. Cranberry Pistachio Vegan Shortbread Cookies 53

28. Garlic Edamame 55

29. Spicy Chickpeas 57

DINNER RECIPES.. 60

30. Avocado Veggie Burritos 61

31. Roasted Squash Gorgonzola Pizza 63

32. Delicious Beef Sirloin Roast.. 65

33. Sweet Seasoned Beef Roast 67

34. Greek Bacon Wrapped Filet Mignon... 69

35. Italian Beef Burgers 71

36. Mexican Beef Jerky 73

37. La Sweet & Spicy Meatballs 75

38. Spiced Seasoned Pork Shoulder.. 77

39. Mexican Seasoned Pork Tenderloin.. 79

40. Air Fryer Garlic Pork Tenderloin... 81

41. Sweetened Pork Tenderloin.. 83

DESSERTS RECIPES.. 86

42. Beignets.. 87

43. S'more 89

44. Fried Oreos... 90

45. Fig Egg Rolls.. 91

46. Grilled Pineapple... 93

47. Chocolate Covered Strawberry S'more..................................... 94

48. Air Fryer Oven Peppermint Lava Cake 95

49.   Air Fryer Oven Chocolate Cake 97

50.   Air Fryer Oven Zucchini Fritters 98

INTRODUCTION

The renal diet has been in use since the middle of the 20th century when the popular scientist discovered some thoughts and conclusions that were healthy and useful for the renal diet. The diet has also improved the health of kidney patients, but it also helps to avoid complications with the kidneys.

Your intake of sodium, protein, potassium and phosphorus is regulated by the Renal Diet. The prevention of renal failure is aided by a renal diet. This is a list of foods/nutrients that should be avoided to prevent kidney problems:

Phosphate: When kidney failure approaches 80 percent and goes to the 4th/5th level of kidney failure, phosphate intake becomes risky. So, by counting the calories and minerals, it is easier to lower your phosphate intake.

Potassium: If your results indicate that your potassium level is elevated in the blood after being diagnosed, then you can reduce your potassium intake. Carrots that are baked and fried are very rich in potassium. Leafy greens, with high levels of potassium in fruit juices. Vegetables low in potassium can still be enjoyed.

Sodium: In our diet, adding salt is very important, but you have to omit or minimize your salt intake when you are suffering from kidney problems. High blood pressure and fluid accumulation in the body can be caused by too much sodium intake. You need to find alternatives that will help season your food. A good choice is herbs and spices that are extracted from plants. Without adding any salt, using garlic, pepper and mustard will improve the taste of your food. Stop sodium-low artificial "salts" because they are rich in potassium, which is also harmful for kidney health.

This cookbook's recipes are plain, tasty, and nutritious. You can also use them to experiment and build your renal diet recipes as an inspiration. It is also possible to see these samples as snacks for you during the day.

A low sodium diet is provided in this cookbook, so knowing the reason for sodium intake is important. Through adding potassium, low sodium consumption, and adding fiber, a low sodium renal diet can be achieved. Many individuals fail to add extra fiber to the diet, and it is viewed as an unhealthy factor many times. But you will soon appreciate the advantages when applied to the renal diet.

You should work with the recipes from this cookbook if you're still used to the renal diet. For more serious and vigilant renal diet beginners, you may use the guide. Try these fast recipes for a better taste if you want to live a happy, safe renal diet!

BREAKFAST RECIPES

1. Spicy Hash Brown Potatoes

Preparation Time: 15 minutes

Cooking Time: 20 minutes

Servings: 4

Ingredients:

- 2 tablespoons chili powder
- 2 teaspoons ground cumin
- 2 teaspoons smoked paprika
- 1 teaspoon garlic powder
- 1 teaspoon cayenne pepper
- 1 teaspoon freshly ground black pepper
- 2 large russet potatoes, peeled
- 2 tablespoons olive oil
- 1/3 cup chopped onion
- 3 garlic cloves, minced
- 1/2 teaspoon sea salt

Directions:

1. For the spice mix: In a small bowl, combine the chili powder, cumin, smoked paprika, garlic powder, cayenne, and black pepper. Transfer to a screw-top glass jar and store in a cool, dry place. (Some of the spice mix is used in this recipe; save the rest for other uses.)

2. Grate the potatoes in a food processor or on the large holes of a box grater. Put the potatoes in a bowl filled with ice water, and let stand for 10 minutes.

3. When the potatoes have soaked, drain them, then dry them well with a kitchen towel.

4. Put the olive oil, onion, and garlic in a 7-inch cake pan.

5. Set or preheat the air fryer to 400°F. Put the onion mixture in the air fryer and cook for 3 minutes, then remove.

6. Put the grated potatoes in a medium bowl and sprinkle with 2 teaspoons of spice mixture and toss. Add to the cake pan with the onion mixture.

7. Cook in the air fryer for 10 minutes, then stir the potatoes gently but thoroughly. Cook for 8 to 12 minutes more or until the potatoes are crisp and light golden brown. Season with salt.

Nutrition: Calories: 235 Total fat: 8g Saturated fat: 1g Cholesterol: 0mg Sodium: 419mg Carbohydrates: 39g Fiber: 5g Protein: 5g

2. Sage and Pear Sausage Patties

Preparation Time: 15 minutes

Cooking Time: 20 minutes

Servings: 6

Ingredients:

- 1pound ground pork
- ¼ cup diced fresh pear
- 1 tablespoon minced fresh sage leaves
- 1 garlic clove, minced
- 1/2 teaspoon sea salt
- 1/8 teaspoon freshly ground black pepper

Directions:

1. In a medium bowl, combine the pork, pear, sage, garlic, salt, and pepper, and mix gently but thoroughly with your hands.
2. Form the mixture into 8 equal patties about 1/2 inch thick.
3. Set or preheat the air fryer to 375°F. Arrange the patties in the air fryer basket in a single layer. You may have to cook the patties in batches.
4. Cook the sausages for 15 to 20 minutes, flipping them halfway through the cooking time, until a meat thermometer registers 160°F. Remove from the air fryer, drain on paper towels for a few minutes, and then serve.

Nutrition: Calories: 204 Total fat: 16g Saturated fat: 6g Cholesterol: 54mg Sodium: 236mg Carbohydrates: 1g Fiber: 0g Protein: 13g

3. Bacon Bombs

Preparation Time: 10 minutes

Cooking Time: 16 minutes

Servings: 4

Ingredients:

- 3 center-cut bacon slices
- 3 large eggs, lightly beaten
- 1 oz 1/3-less-fat cream cheese, softened
- 1 tbsp chopped fresh chives
- 4 oz fresh whole wheat pizza dough
- Cooking spray

Directions:

1. Sear the bacon slices in a skillet until brown and crispy then chop into fine crumbles. Add eggs to the same pan and cook for 1 minute then stir in cream cheese, chives and bacon. Mix well, then allow this egg filling to cool down. Spread the pizza dough and slice into four -5inches circles. Divide the egg filling on top of each circle and seal its edge to make dumplings. Place the bacon bombs in the Air Fryer basket and spray them with cooking oil. Set the Air Fryer basket inside the Air Fryer toaster oven and close the lid. Select the Air Fry mode at 350 degrees F temperature for 6 minutes. Serve warm.

Nutrition: Calories: 278 Protein: 7.9g Carbs: 23g Fat: 3.9g

4. Morning Potatoes

Preparation Time: 10 minutes

Cooking Time: 23 minutes

Servings: 4

Ingredients:

- 2 russet potatoes, washed & diced
- 1/2 tsp salt
- 1 tbsp. olive oil
- ¼ tsp garlic powder
- Chopped parsley, for garnish

Directions:

1. Soak the potatoes in cold water for 45 minutes, then drain and dry them. Toss potato cubes with garlic powder, salt, and olive oil in the Air Fryer basket. Set the Air Fryer basket inside the Air Fryer toaster oven and close the lid. Select the Air Fry mode at 400 degrees F temperature for 23 minutes. Toss them well when cooked halfway through then continue cooking. Garnish with chopped parsley to serve.

Nutrition: Calories: 146 Protein: 6.2g Carbs: 41.2g Fat: 5g

5. Breakfast Pockets

Preparation Time: 10 minutes

Cooking Time: 10 minutes

Servings: 6

Ingredients:

- 1 box puff pastry sheet
- 5 eggs
- 1/2 cup loose sausage, cooked
- 1/2 cup bacon, cooked
- 1/2 cup cheddar cheese, shredded

Directions:

2. Stir cook egg in a skillet for 1 minute then mix with sausages, cheddar cheese, and bacon. Spread the pastry sheet and cut it into four rectangles of equal size.
3. Divide the egg mixture over each rectangle. Fold the edges around the filling and seal them. Place the pockets in the Air Fryer basket.
4. Set the Air Fryer basket inside the Air Fryer toaster oven and close the lid. Select the Air Fry mode at 370 degrees F temperature for 10 minutes. Serve warm.

Nutrition: Calories: 387 Protein: 14.6g Carbs: 37.4g Fat: 6g

6. Avocado Flautas

Preparation Time: 10 minutes

Cooking Time: 24 minutes

Servings: 8

Ingredients:

- 1 tbsp butter
- 8 eggs, beaten
- 1/2 tsp salt
- ¼ tsp pepper
- 1 1/2 tsp cumin
- 1 tsp chili powder
- 8 fajita-size tortillas
- 4 oz cream cheese, softened
- 8 slices cooked bacon
- Avocado Crème:
- 2 small avocados
- 1/2 cup sour cream
- 1 lime, juiced
- 1/2 tsp salt
- ¼ tsp pepper

Directions:

1. In a skillet, melt butter and stir in eggs, salt, cumin, pepper, and chili powder, then stir cook for 4 minutes. Spread all the tortillas and top them with cream cheese and bacon. Then

divide the egg scramble on top and finally add cheese. Roll the tortillas to seal the filling inside. Place 4 rolls in the Air Fryer basket. Set the Air Fryer basket inside the Air Fryer toaster oven and close the lid. Select the Air Fry mode at 400 degrees F temperature for 12 minutes. Cook the remaining tortilla rolls in the same manner. Meanwhile, blend avocado crème ingredients in a blender then serves with warm flautas.

Nutrition: Calories: 212 Protein: 17.3g Carbs: 14.6g Fat: 11.8g

7. Cheese Sandwiches

Preparation Time: 10 minutes

Cooking Time: 10 minutes

Servings: 2

Ingredients:

- 1 egg
- 3 tbsp half and half cream
- ¼ tsp vanilla extract
- 2 slices sourdough, white or multigrain bread
- 21/2 oz sliced Swiss cheese
- 2 oz sliced deli ham
- 2 oz sliced deli turkey
- 1 tsp butter, melted
- Powdered sugar
- Raspberry jam, for serving

Directions:

1. Beat egg with half and half cream and vanilla extract in a bowl. Place one bread slice on the working surface and top it with ham and turkey slice and swiss cheese.

2. Place the other bread slice on top, then dip the sandwich in the egg mixture, then place it in a suitable baking tray lined with butter.

3. Set the baking tray inside the Air Fryer toaster oven and close the lid. Select the Air Fry mode at 350 degrees F temperature for 10 minutes. Flip the sandwich and continue cooking for 8 minutes. Slice and serve.

Nutrition: Calories: 412 Protein: 18.9g Carbs: 43.8g Fat: 24.8g

8. Sausage Cheese Wraps

Preparation Time: 10 minutes

Cooking Time: 3 minutes

Servings: 8

Ingredients:

- 8 sausages
- 2 pieces American cheese, shredded
- 8-count refrigerated crescent roll dough

Directions:

1. Roll out each crescent roll and top it with cheese and 1 sausage. Fold both the top and bottom edges of the crescent sheet to cover the sausage and roll it around the sausage. Place 4 rolls in the Air Fryer basket and spray them with cooking oil. Set the Air Fryer basket inside the Air Fryer toaster oven and close the lid. Select the Air Fry mode at 380 degrees F temperature for 3 minutes. Cook the remaining rolls in the same manner. Serve fresh.

Nutrition: Calories: 296 Protein: 34.2gC Carbs: 17g Fat: 22.1g

9. Sausage Burritos

Preparation Time: 10 minutes

Cooking Time: 10 minutes

Servings: 6

Ingredients:

- 6 medium flour tortillas
- 6 scrambled eggs
- 1/2 lb. ground sausage, browned
- 1/2 bell pepper, minced
- 1/3 cup bacon bits
- 1/2 cup shredded cheese
- Oil, for spraying

Directions:

2. Mix eggs with cheese, bell pepper, bacon, and sausage in a bowl. Spread each tortilla on the working surface and top it with 1/2 cup egg filling.

3. Roll the tortilla like a burrito then place 3 burritos in the Air Fryer basket. Spray them with cooking oil.

4. Set the Air Fryer basket inside the Air Fryer toaster oven and close the lid. Select the Air Fry mode at 330 degrees F temperature for 5 minutes. Cook the remaining burritos in the same manner. Serve fresh.

Nutrition: Calories: 197 Protein: 7.9g Carbs: 58.5g Fat: 15.4g

10. Sausage Patties

Preparation Time: 10 minutes

Cooking Time: 20 minutes

Servings: 4

Ingredients:

- lbs. ground sausage
- 1 tsp chili flakes
- 1 tsp dried thyme
- 1 tsp onion powder
- 1/2 tsp each paprika and cayenne
- Sea salt and black pepper, to taste
- 2 tsp brown sugar
- 3 tsp minced garlic
- 2 tsp Tabasco
- Herbs for garnish

Directions:

1. Toss sausage ground with all the spices, herbs, sugar, garlic and tabasco sauce in a bowl. Make 1.5-inch-thick and 3-inch round patties out of this mixture. Place the sausage patties in the Air Fryer basket. Set the Air Fryer basket inside the Air Fryer toaster oven and close the lid. Select the Air Fry mode at 370 degrees F temperature for 20 minutes. Flip the patties when cooked halfway through then continue cooking.

Nutrition: Calories: 208 Protein: 24.3g Carbs: 9.5g Fat: 10.7g

11. Spicy Sweet Potato Hash

Preparation Time: 10 minutes

Cooking Time: 16 minutes

Servings: 4

Ingredients:

- 2 large sweet potato, diced
- 2 slices bacon, cooked and diced
- 2 tbsp olive oil
- 1 tbsp smoked paprika
- 1 tsp of sea salt
- 1 tsp ground black pepper
- 1 tsp dried dill weed

Directions:

1. Toss sweet potato with all the spices and olive oil in the Air Fry basket. Set the Air Fryer basket inside the Air Fryer toaster oven and close the lid. Select the Air Fry mode at 400 degrees F temperature for 16 minutes. Toss the potatoes after every 5 minutes. Once done, toss in bacon and serve warm.

Nutrition: Calories: 134 Protein: 6.6g Carbs: 36.5g Fat: 6g

LUNCH RECIPES

12. Olives and Zucchini Cakes

Preparation Time: 17 minutes

Cooking Time: 6 minutes

Servings: 6

Ingredients:

- 3spring onions; chopped.

- 1/2 cup kalamata olives, pitted and minced

- 3zucchinis; grated

- 1/2 cup parsley; chopped.

- 1/2 cup almond flour

- 1egg

- Cooking spray

- Salt and black pepper to taste.

Directions:

1. Take a bowl and mix all the ingredients except the cooking spray, stir well and shape medium cakes out of this mixture

2. Place the cakes in your air fryer's basket, grease them with cooking spray and cook at 380°F for 6 minutes on each side. Serve as an appetizer.

Nutrition: Calories: 165 Fat: 5g Fiber: 2g Carbs: 3g Protein: 7g

13. Fluffy Strawberry Muffins

Preparation Time: 10 minutes

Cooking Time: 25 minutes

Servings: 12

Ingredients:

- 1 1/2 cups almond flour
- 1 tsp baking powder
- 1/2 tsp xanthan gum
- 1/2 cup Lakanto monk fruit sweetener
- 2 eggs, beaten
- 1 tsp vanilla extract
- 1/2 tsp almond extract
- 3 tbsps. Unsalted butter
- 3 tbsps. Unsweetened vanilla almond milk
- 1/2 cup chopped strawberries

Directions:

1. Preheat the oven to 350° F.
2. Take the 2 eggs and beat them with vanilla extract, melted butter, almond extract, and unsweetened almond milk until creamy and smooth. This should take around 2 minutes.
3. In another bowl, mix sweetener, xanthan gum, baking powder, and almond flour.
4. Combine the dry and wet ingredients and mix well; you should not have any lumps.

5. Add the chopped strawberries to the batter and use a plastic spatula to fold them in.

6. Take a muffin tin and put cupcake liners in each of the molds. Fill ¾ of each mold with the batter.

7. Bake for 20-25 minutes. You can check if they are done by inserting a toothpick into the center of a muffin; the toothpick will come out clean if they are done.

Nutrition: Calories 144 Carbs 2g Protein 5g Fat 13g Fiber 2g

14. Paleo Blueberry Muffins

Preparation Time: 10 minutes

Cooking Time: 20 minutes

Servings: 12

Ingredients:

- 1/2 cup coconut flour
- 4 1/2 tbsps. coconut oil
- 6 organic eggs
- 4 tbsps. milk
- 1/2 tsp apple cider vinegar
- 1/2 tsp baking soda
- ¼ tsp baking powder
- 1 tsp cinnamon
- ¼ tsp sea salt
- 2 tbsps. raw honey
- 1/2 cup blueberries

Directions:

1. Preheat the oven to 400° F.
2. Combine all wet ingredients (coconut oil, eggs, milk, apple cider vinegar, honey) in a medium-sized bowl.
3. In another bowl, mix all the dry ingredients (coconut flour, baking soda, baking powder, cinnamon, sea salt).
4. Add dry ingredients to the bowl of the wet ingredients and combine them well.

5. Add blueberries to the batter and stir thoroughly. The blueberries should be evenly spread throughout the batter.

6. Pour batter into baking cups or a muffin tin. If you are using a muffin tin, make sure to use cupcake liners.

7. Bake for 10-15 minutes, or until golden brown.

Nutrition: Calories 210 Carbs 6g Sugar 2g Protein 7g Fat 19g Fiber 3g

15. Orange Cardamom Muffins with Coconut Butter Glaze

Preparation Time: 10 minutes

Cooking Time: 30 minutes

Servings: 6

Ingredients:

- 2 cups blanched almond flour
- 3 large eggs
- 1 tbsp orange zest
- ¼ cup fresh orange juice
- 1/2 tsp cardamom
- ¼ tsp salt
- 1 tsp baking powder
- 2 tsp Stevia sweetener
- 2 tbsps. Coconut oil, melted
- For coconut butter glaze:
- 1 tbsp coconut oil
- ¼ cup coconut butter
- 1/2 tbsp Stevia sweetener

Directions:

1. Preheat the oven to 350° F.
2. In a medium-sized bowl, whisk eggs, orange zest, and orange juice.

3. In another bowl, combine the dry ingredients (almond flour, cardamom, salt, baking powder, and sweetener).

4. Combine dry ingredients with the wet ingredients by folding them in gently, then stir to form an even better.

5. After this, add the coconut oil and fold through again.

6. Line muffin tin with paper liners and pour 1/3 cup of batter into each muffin cup.

7. Bake for 25-30 minutes.

8. When done, let the cupcakes cool down for at least 10 minutes.

9. While your cupcakes are cooling, start working on the glaze. Start by melting the coconut oil and coconut butter on the stove.

10. Stir this mixture until it is smooth and take it off the stove, then add the sweetener.

11. Once your cupcakes have fully cooled, drizzle the glaze on top of them.

Nutrition: Calories 219 Carbs 7g Sugar 2g Protein 5.5g Fat 20g Fiber 2.5g

16. Bacon and Egg Cups

Preparation Time: 10 minutes

Cooking Time: 20 minutes

Servings: 6

Ingredients:

- 6 eggs
- 2 tbsps. fresh parsley
- 3 ounces of cheddar cheese
- 6 slices regular-cut bacon
- Salt and pepper to taste

Directions:

1. Preheat the oven to 350° F.
2. Spray or grease your muffin pan with coconut oil.
3. Line the sides of each muffin cup with a bacon slice.
4. Crack an egg into each bacon-lined muffin cup.
5. Add salt and pepper, and sprinkle with cheese.
6. Bake for 20 minutes; the eggs need this much time to cook fully.
7. Garnish with chopped parsley and serve.

Nutrition: Calories 210 Carbs 0g Sugar 0g   Protein 15g Fat 16g

17. Breadsticks

Preparation Time: 20 minutes

Cooking Time: 10 minutes

Servings: 12

Ingredients:

- 1 1/2 cups part skim low moisture shredded mozzarella cheese
- 1 ounce of cream cheese
- 1/2 cup almond flour
- 3 tbsps. Coconut flour
- 1 large egg
- For topping:
- 1/2 cup part skim low moisture shredded mozzarella cheese
- 1/2 cup shredded Parmesan cheese
- 1 tsp finely chopped parsley

Directions:

1. Preheat the oven to 425° F.
2. Melt the cheese you will use in your batter. Put the cream cheese and mozzarella in a microwaveable bowl and microwave for 1 minute. Stir, then put it back in for another 30 seconds. Keep repeating this process until you end up with a smooth and even mixture.

3. Use a food processor on a high speed to combine the cheese mixture with coconut flour, almond flour, and egg. The end result should be a uniform mixture without any lumps.

4. The dough will be a little sticky at this stage and will need to cool down a bit. Cooling the dough will help you roll it out easier.

5. Between 2 pieces of parchment paper, roll the dough to around ¼ inch thick, then remove top piece of parchment paper.

6. Transfer dough and parchment paper to a baking sheet and spread ¼ cup mozzarella cheese over the top of the dough.

7. Bake for 5-6 minutes, or until the edges are golden and puffy.

8. Sprinkle Parmesan cheese and the rest of the mozzarella on the dough and bake for another 4-5 minutes, or until cheese is melted.

9. Once baked, garnish with parsley and serve.

Nutrition: Calories 207 Carbs 7g Sugar 2gProtein 13g Fat 14g

18. Butter Crackers

Preparation Time: 5 minutes

Cooking Time: 15 minutes

Servings: 25

Ingredients:

- 8 tbsps. Salted butter, softened
- 2 egg whites
- 2 ¼ cups almond flour
- Salt to taste

Directions:

1. Preheat the oven to 350° F.
2. Combine butter and almond flour in a medium bowl and mix on low-medium speed with an electric mixer.
3. Add egg whites and salt to this mixture and combine them with the mixer. You should expect to have smooth dough within 5-10 minutes.
4. Roll the dough between 2 pieces of parchment paper to a thickness of around 1/8 inch.
5. Remove the top parchment paper and place the dough and bottom parchment paper onto the baking sheet.
6. Use a pizza cutter or knife to divide the dough into 2-inch squares. You can sprinkle the dough with salt if you prefer.
7. Bake for 10-15 minutes, or until golden brown; the time will vary according to the width of the dough squares.

8. Serve immediately, while they are still crunchy. However, if you want to store them, keep them in an airtight container rather than in the refrigerator; the refrigerator causes the crackers to lose their crunch.

Nutrition: Calories 90 Carbs 8g Protein 2g Fat 8g Fiber 1g

19. Homemade Almond Crackers

Preparation Time: 15 minutes

Cooking Time: 30 minutes

Servings: 12

Ingredients:

- 1 cup almond flour
- 3 tbsps. Water
- 1 tbsp ground flaxseed
- 1/2 tsp fine sea salt
- Flaked sea salt to garnish (optional)

Directions:

1. Preheat the oven to 350° F.
2. Combine almond flour, water, ground flaxseed, and salt in a large bowl and stir the mixture to form dough.
3. Place the dough between 2 pieces of parchment paper and roll it to 1/8 inch thick.
4. Dispose of top piece of parchment paper, then sprinkle flaked sea salt on the dough. Press the salt into the dough with your fingers.
5. With a knife, cut the dough into small 1-inch by 1-inch squares. You can also use a toothpick to create little holes in the crackers.
6. Place the parchment paper with the dough pieces into the oven and bake for 25-30 minutes, or until golden brown.

7. Allow the crackers to cool down before serving. If you are not eating them immediately, make sure to use an airtight container to store them.

Nutrition: Calories 173 Carbs 7g Sugar 1g Protein 6gFat 15g Fiber 4g

20. Pepperoni Chips

Preparation Time: 2 minutes

Cooking Time: 6 minutes

Servings: 6

Ingredients:

- 6 ounces of pepperoni

Directions:

1. Preheat the oven to 400° F.

2. Thinly slice the pepperoni.

3. Place a piece of parchment paper on a baking sheet, then place all the pepperoni slices at an equal distance from each other on the sheet.

4. Bake for 5 minutes, then use a power towel to sponge off the excess oil from the slices.

5. To crisp them up, put the slices back in the oven for 1 more minute. However, depending on how crisp you want them to be, you can keep them in for a bit longer. Remember, don't burn them!

6. Let them cool before serving.

Nutrition: Calories 140 Carbs 0g Sugar 0g Protein 5g Fat 12g

21. 3-Ingredient Flourless Cheesy Breadsticks

Preparation Time: 15 minutes

Cooking Time: 25 minutes

Servings: 10

Ingredients:

- 1 1/2 cups shredded mozzarella cheese
- 2 large eggs
- 1/2 tsp Italian seasoning
- For topping:
- 1/2 cup shredded mozzarella cheese
- 2 tbsps. Shredded parmesan cheese (optional)
- 1 tsp finely chopped parsley (optional)

Directions:

1. Preheat the oven to 350° F.
2. Line a 9-inch by 9-inch baking pan with parchment paper.
3. Blend the eggs and shredded mozzarella cheese until everything is combined evenly. Add Italian seasoning at this stage. An electric mixer is recommended.
4. Mixture needs to be evenly spread out in the baking pan and baked for 20 minutes. Once done, the crust should be firm.
5. Allow it to cool for at least 5 minutes.
6. Increase oven temperature to 425° F.
7. Remove crust from parchment paper and place it on a cooling rack. Add the remaining cheese on top of the crust. You can

use parmesan or cheddar instead of mozzarella, depending on what you prefer.

8. Bake crust on cooling rack in oven for about 5 more minutes so it crisps up.

9. Garnish with parsley, then serve.

Nutrition: Calories 142 Carbs 3g Sugar 1g Protein 11g Fat 9g

22. Cauliflower Breadsticks

Preparation Time: 10 minutes

Cooking Time: 32 minutes

Servings: 8-10

Ingredients:

- 2 cups cauliflower rice
- 2 eggs
- 1/2 tsp granulated garlic
- 1/2 tsp ground pepper
- 1 cup shredded mozzarella or Mexican blend cheese
- ¼ cup grated Parmesan cheese
- 1 tsp Italian Seasoning
- 1/2 tsp salt

Directions:

1. Preheat the oven to 350° F.
2. Grease a baking sheet with oil or butter. If you are not greasing, then remember to place a piece of parchment paper on the baking sheet.
3. Combine cauliflower rice, eggs, garlic, pepper, and cheese to a food processor. Add salt and Italian seasoning at this stage. Work at low or medium speeds to break down the cauliflower as much as possible so that a smooth mixture is formed.
4. Pour mixture onto the baking sheet. The dough should have a thickness of around ¼ inch.

5. Bake for 30 minutes.

6. Add more cheese on top after you have taken it out of the oven.

7. Bake for another 2-3 minutes to melt the added cheese.

8. Cut into 8-10 breadstick slices and serve.

Nutrition: Calories 165 Carbs 5g Sugar 1g Protein 13g Fat 10g

23. Breadsticks with Mozzarella Dough

Preparation Time: 10 minutes

Cooking Time: 10 minutes

Servings: 10

Ingredients:

- 2/3 cup almond flour
- 1 ¾ cups shredded mozzarella cheese
- 2 tbsps. Full-fat cream cheese
- Pinch of salt to taste
- 1 medium egg
- 1 tbsp garlic, crushed
- 1 tsp dried rosemary
- 1 tbsp parsley, fresh or dried

Directions:

1. Preheat the oven to 425° F.
2. In a large microwavable bowl, combine almond flour, mozzarella, cream cheese, and salt, and microwave for 1 minute.
3. Stir the mixture and microwave for another 30 seconds.
4. Add the egg to create a cheesy dough.
5. Make dough balls and roll them into long, thin breadsticks. The smaller the dough balls, the more breadsticks you will be able to make.

6. Bake for 10 minutes, or until golden brown. Check after 5 minutes and see whether they are golden brown or not. If they are too light, put them back into the oven for another 5 minutes. If they are already done, take them out. The baking time can vary depending on the thickness of the breadsticks.

Nutrition: Calories 58 Carbs 1.2 g Sugar 0.3g Protein 2g Fat 5g Fiber 0.5g

24. Bacon Onion Cookies

Preparation Time: 15 minutes

Cooking Time: 15 minutes

Servings: 12

Ingredients:

- 4 slices bacon, crisped and crumbled
- 1 tbsp onion powder
- 1/2 tsp sea salt or pink Himalayan rock salt
- Pinch of freshly ground pepper
- 1 1/2 cups almond flour
- 1 tbsp psyllium husk powder
- 1/3 cup flax meal
- 1 large egg

Directions:

1. Preheat the oven to 375° F.
2. Put a piece of parchment paper on a baking sheet. Carefully line the bacon slices on the sheet and put it in the oven for around 10 minutes, or until it reaches your preferred crispiness.
3. In a bowl, mix onion powder, salt, pepper, almond flour, psyllium husk powder, and flax meal.
4. Add the egg to the dry ingredients and work the dough with your hands.
5. Crumble your bacon slices and add them to the dough.

6. Put a fresh piece of parchment paper on your baking sheet.

7. Form small or medium dough balls and space them equally on your baking sheet.

8. Use a fork to press the dough balls down and flatten them.

9. Bake for 10-12 minutes, or until golden brown. Keep a close eye on the cookies as they bake since almond flour can burn easily.

10. Cool before serving. Use an airtight container for storage.

Nutrition: Calories 109 Carbs 4.3 g Protein 4.8 g Fat 9g Fiber 2.7 g

25. Cinnamon Swirl Cookies

Preparation Time: 30 minutes

Cooking Time: 50 minutes

Servings: 8

Ingredients:

- 3 cups almond flour
- 1/2 cup low-carb sweetener
- 2 tsps. gluten-free baking powder
- ¼ tsp salt
- 1 egg
- 2 tbsps. butter, melted
- 2 tsps. cinnamon

Directions:

1. In a large bowl, mix almond flour, sweetener, baking powder, and salt.
2. Add butter and egg to the dry ingredients. You will see the dough forming as you mix and combine.
3. Divide the dough into 2 equal parts. Add cinnamon to one and leave the other one plain.
4. Keep both doughs in the bowl and cover with plastic wrap or a kitchen towel. Put in the refrigerator for at least 30 minutes.
5. Preheat the oven to 280° F.
6. Roll both types of dough to ¼ inch thick between 2 pieces of parchment paper.

7. Place cinnamon dough on top of plain dough and roll into a tight log.

8. Cut dough log into cookies that are about 1/2 inch thick.

9. Place cookies on a baking sheet lined with parchment paper and bake for 30 minutes, or until golden brown.

10. Cool before serving.

Nutrition: Nutrition Facts Serving size: 1 cookie Calories 106 Carbs 2g Sugar 1g Protein 4g Fat 9g Fiber 2g

26. Peanut Butter Cookies

Preparation Time: 5 minutes

Cooking Time: 15 minutes

Servings: 12

Ingredients:

- 1/2 cup peanut butter
- ¼ cup powdered erythritol sweetener
- 1 egg

Directions:

1. Preheat the oven to 350° F.
2. Use a spatula to combine peanut butter, powdered sweetener, and egg.
3. Use a cookie scoop to scoop cookie dough into balls of a uniform size.
4. Line a baking sheet with parchment paper and place the cookie dough balls on it in a vertical line.
5. Bake for 12-15 minutes, or until crisp and golden brown.
6. Cool for at least 10 minutes before serving.

Nutrition: Calories 82 Carbs 3g Protein 4gFat 7gFiber 1g

27. Cranberry Pistachio Vegan Shortbread Cookies

Preparation Time: 20 minutes

Cooking Time: 10 minutes

Servings: 12

Ingredients:

- 2 cups ground almond flour
- 1/3 cup coconut sugar
- 1/2 tsp baking soda
- 1/2 tsp sea salt
- 1/2 cup pistachios, shelled and chopped
- 1/2 cup dried cranberries
- 1/2 cup coconut oil
- For dipping the cookies (optional):
- 2/3 cup chocolate chips

Directions:

1. Use a mixer to combine all the ingredientsfor the shortbread. Keep beating until a crumbly dough has formed.
2. Place the dough onto a piece of plastic wrap and shape it into a cylinder.
3. Wrap the dough in plastic wrap and put it into the freezer for a minimum of 2 hours. When you are ready to bake it, let it thaw for a little bit; chilling the dough makes it easier to cut when you are ready.

4. Preheat the oven to 350° F and line a baking sheet with parchment paper.
5. Use a knife to cut the dough into ¼-inch to 1/2-inch thick disks and lay these on the parchment paper.
6. Bake the cookies for 10-15 minutes, or until golden brown.
7. Let them cool for at least 30 minutes.
8. If you want to drizzle chocolate on your cookies or dip them in chocolate, melt the chocolate chips in the microwave for 10 seconds. Stir chocolate and repeat until it has reached a smooth consistency.

Nutrition: Calories 192 Carbs 13g Sugar 11g Protein 2g Fat 15.5g Fiber 1g

28. Garlic Edamame

Preparation Time: 5 minutes

Cooking Time: 10 minutes

Servings: 4

Ingredients:

- Olive oil
- 1 (16-ounce) bag frozen edamame in pods
- 1/2 teaspoon salt
- 1/2 teaspoon garlic salt
- ¼ teaspoon freshly ground black pepper
- 1/2 teaspoon red pepper flakes (optional)

Directions:

1. Spray a fryer basket lightly with olive oil.
2. In a medium bowl, add the frozen edamame and lightly spray with olive oil. Toss to coat.
3. In a small bowl, mix together the salt, garlic salt, black pepper, and red pepper flakes (if using). Add the mixture to the edamame and toss until evenly coated.
4. Place half the edamame in the fryer basket. Do not overfill the basket.
5. Air fry for 5 minutes. Shake the basket and cook until the edamame is starting to brown and get crispy, 3 to 5 more minutes.
6. Repeat with the remaining edamame and serve immediately.
7. Pair It With: These make a nice side dish to almost any meal.

8. Air Fry Like a Pro: If you use fresh edamame, reduce the air fry time by 2 to 3 minutes to avoid overcooking. Air-fried edamame do not retain their crisp texture, so it's best to eat them right after cooking.

Nutrition: Calories: 100 Total Fat: 3g Saturated Fat: 0g Cholesterol: 0mg Carbohydrates: 9g Protein: 8g Fiber: 4g Sodium: 496mg

29. Spicy Chickpeas

Preparation Time: 5 minutes

Cooking Time: 20 minutes

Servings: 4

Ingredients:

- Olive oil
- 1/2 teaspoon ground cumin
- 1/2 teaspoon chili powder
- ¼ teaspoon cayenne pepper
- ¼ teaspoon salt
- 1 (19-ounce) can chickpeas, drained and rinsed

Directions:

1. Spray a fryer basket lightly with olive oil.
2. In a small bowl, combine the cumin, chili powder, cayenne pepper, and salt.
3. In a medium bowl, add the chickpeas and lightly spray them with olive oil. Add the spice mixture and toss until coated evenly.
4. Transfer the chickpeas to the fryer basket. Air fry until the chickpeas reach your desired level of crunchiness, 15 to 20 minutes, making sure to shake the basket every 5 minutes.
5. Air Fry Like a Pro: I find 20 minutes to be the sweet spot for very crunchy chickpeas. If you prefer them less crispy, cook for about 15 minutes. These make a great vehicle for experimenting with different seasoning mixes such as Chinese

5-spice, a mixture of curry and turmeric, or herbes de Provence.

Nutrition: Calories: 122 Total Fat: 1g Saturated Fat: 0g Cholesterol: 0mg Carbohydrates: 22g Protein: 6g Fiber: 6g Sodium: 152mg

DINNER RECIPES

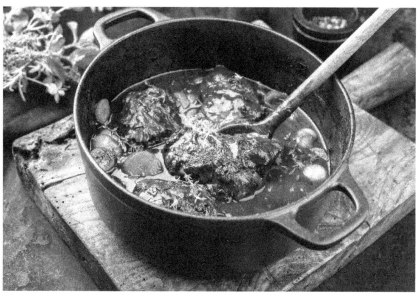

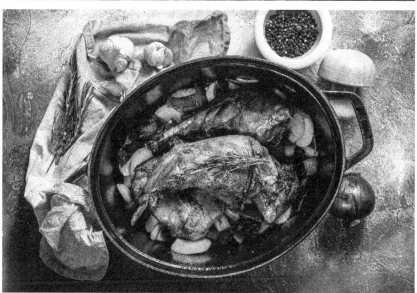

30. Avocado Veggie Burritos

Preparation Time: 15 minutes

Cooking Time: 6 minutes, plus 12 minutes to heat if desired

Servings: 4

Ingredients:

- 1 onion, chopped
- 1 red bell pepper, chopped
- 1 tablespoon olive oil
- 3 plum tomatoes, seeded and chopped
- 1 cup frozen corn kernels, thawed
- 2 teaspoons chili powder
- 1/2 teaspoon sea salt
- 1/8 Teaspoon freshly ground black pepper
- 1 avocado, flesh removed
- 1 tablespoon freshly squeezed lemon juice
- 4 (8-inch) flour tortillas
- 11/2 cups shredded pepper Jack cheese

Directions:

1. Combine the onion and red bell pepper in the air fryer basket. Drizzle with the olive oil and toss to coat.

2. Set or preheat the air fryer to 375°F. Roast 4 to 6 minutes, or until the vegetables are tender. Transfer the vegetables to a medium bowl; let the air fryer basket cool for 10 minutes, then rinse out the basket and dry it.

3. Put the tomatoes, corn, chili powder, salt, and pepper in the bowl and mix to combine.

4. In a small bowl, mash the avocado with the lemon juice.

5. Warm the tortillas according to the package directions.

6. Put the tortillas on a work surface. Spread each with the avocado mixture and sprinkle with the cheese. Top with the vegetable mixture.

7. Fold up the bottoms of the tortillas, then fold in the sides and roll up, enclosing the filling.

8. At this point you can serve the burritos as-is or heat them until they are crisp.

9. To heat, set or preheat the air fryer to 375°F. Seal the burritos with a toothpick if necessary. Then place the burritos, seam-side down, in the basket; mist with cooking oil. Bake for 5 minutes, then turn over carefully, mist with oil again, and bake for 4 to 7 minutes more until crisp. Serve.

Nutrition: Calories 491 Protein 18g Fat 28g Saturated Fat 11g Carbs 46g

31. Roasted Squash Gorgonzola Pizza

Preparation Time: 10 minutes

Cooking Time: 42 minutes

Servings: 4

Ingredients:

- 1 (16-ounce) package cubed fresh butternut squash
- 2 tablespoons olive oil
- 1/2 teaspoon sea salt
- 1/8 Teaspoon freshly ground black pepper
- 1 (8-ounce) package cream cheese, at room temperature
- 2 tablespoons sour cream
- 2 (8-inch) round focaccia breads
- 2/3 Cup crumbled gorgonzola cheese

Directions:

1. Place the squash in the air fryer basket, drizzle with the olive oil, and sprinkle with the salt and pepper. Toss to coat.

2. Set or preheat the air fryer to 400°F. Roast for 15 to 20 minutes, tossing once halfway through cooking time, until the squash is tender and light brown around the edges.

3. Transfer to a bowl. Clean the air fryer basket before you start the pizzas.

4. In a small bowl, combine the cream cheese and sour cream and beat until smooth. Spread this mixture onto the focaccia breads.

5. Divide the roasted squash and the gorgonzola between the two pizzas. Working in batches, place one pizza in the air fryer basket.

6. Set or preheat the air fryer to 400°F. Bake for 7 to 11 minutes or until the crust is crisp and the pizza is hot. Repeat with remaining pizza. Serve hot.

Nutrition: Calories 441 Protein 13g Fat 29g Saturated Fat 15g Carbs 32g

32. Delicious Beef Sirloin Roast

Preparation Time: 10 minutes

Cooking Time: 50 minutes

Servings: 8

Ingredients:

- 21/2 pounds sirloin roast
- Salt and ground black pepper, as required

Directions:

1. Rub the roast with salt and black pepper generously.
2. Insert the rotisserie rod through the roast.
3. Insert the rotisserie forks, one on each side of the rod to secure the rod to the chicken.
4. Arrange the drip pan in the bottom of Instant Vortex Plus Air Fryer Oven cooking chamber.
5. Select "Roast" and then adjust the temperature to 350 degrees F.
6. Set the timer for 50 minutes and press the "Start".
7. When the display shows "Add Food" press the red lever down and load the left side of the rod into the Vortex.
8. Now, slide the rod's left side into the groove along the metal bar so it doesn't move.
9. Then, close the door and touch "Rotate".
10. When cooking time is complete, press the red lever to release the rod.

11. Remove from the Vortex and place the roast onto a platter for about 10 minutes before slicing.

12. With a sharp knife, cut the roast into desired sized slices and serve.

Nutrition: Calories 201 Total Fat 8.8 g Saturated Fat 3.1 g Cholesterol 94 mg Sodium 88 mg Protein 28.9 g

33. Sweet Seasoned Beef Roast

Preparation Time: 10 minutes

Cooking Time: 45 minutes

Servings: 10

Ingredients:

- 3 pounds beef top roast
- 1 tablespoon olive oil
- 2 tablespoons Montreal steak seasoning

Directions:

1. Coat the roast with oil and then rub with the seasoning generously.
2. With kitchen twines, tie the roast to keep it compact.
3. Arrange the roast onto the cooking tray.
4. Arrange the drip pan in the bottom of Instant Vortex plus Air Fryer Oven cooking chamber.
5. Select "Air Fry" and then adjust the temperature to 360 degrees F.
6. Set the timer for 45 minutes and press the "Start".
7. When the display shows "Add Food" insert the cooking tray in the center position.
8. When the display shows "Turn Food" do nothing.
9. When cooking time is complete, remove the tray from Vortex and place the roast onto a platter for about 10 minutes before slicing.

10. With a sharp knife, cut the roast into desired sized slices and serve.

Nutrition: Calories 269 Total Fat 9.9 g Saturated Fat 3.4 g Cholesterol 122 mg Sodium 538 mg Protein 41.3 g

34. Greek Bacon Wrapped Filet Mignon

Preparation Time: 10 minutes

Cooking Time: 15 minutes

Servings: 2

Ingredients:

- 2 bacon slices
- 2 (4-ounce) filet mignon
- Salt and ground black pepper, as required
- Olive oil cooking spray

Directions:

1. Wrap 1 bacon slice around each filet mignon and secure with toothpicks.
2. Season the filets with the salt and black pepper lightly.
3. Arrange the filet mignon onto a coking rack and spray with cooking spray.
4. Arrange the drip pan in the bottom of Instant Vortex plus Air Fryer Oven cooking chamber.
5. Select "Air Fry" and then adjust the temperature to 375 degrees F.
6. Set the timer for 15 minutes and press the "Start".
7. When the display shows "Add Food" insert the cooking rack in the center position.
8. When the display shows "Turn Food" turn the filets.
9. When cooking time is complete, remove the rack from Vortex and serve hot.

Nutrition: Calories 360 Total Fat 19.6 g Saturated Fat 6.8 g Cholesterol 108 mg Sodium 737 mg Protein 42.6 g

35. Italian Beef Burgers

Preparation Time: 15 minutes

Cooking Time: 18 minutes

Servings: 4

Ingredients:

- For Burgers:
- 1-pound ground beef
- 1/2 cup panko breadcrumbs
- ¼ cup onion, chopped finely
- 3 tablespoons Dijon mustard
- 3 teaspoons low-sodium soy sauce
- 2 teaspoons fresh rosemary, chopped finely
- Salt, to taste
- For Topping:
- 2 tablespoons Dijon mustard
- 1 tablespoon brown sugar
- 1 teaspoon soy sauce
- 4 Gruyere cheese slices

Directions:

1. In a large bowl, add all the ingredients and mix until well combined.
2. Make 4 equal-sized patties from the mixture.
3. Arrange the patties onto a cooking tray.

4. Arrange the drip pan in the bottom of Instant Vortex plus Air Fryer Oven cooking chamber.

5. Select "Air Fry" and then adjust the temperature to 370 degrees F.

6. Set the timer for 15 minutes and press the "Start".

7. When the display shows "Add Food" insert the cooking rack in the center position.

8. When the display shows "Turn Food" turn the burgers.

9. Meanwhile, for sauce: in a small bowl, add the mustard, brown sugar and soy sauce and mix well.

10. When cooking time is complete, remove the tray from Vortex and coat the burgers with the sauce.

11. Top each burger with 1 cheese slice.

12. Return the tray to the cooking chamber and select "Broil".

13. Set the timer for 3 minutes and press the "Start".

14. When cooking time is complete, remove the tray from Vortex and serve hot.

Nutrition: Calories 402 Total Fat 18 g Saturated Fat 8.5 g Cholesterol 133mg Sodium 651 mg Total Carbs 6.3 g Fiber 0.8 g Sugar 3 g Protein 44.4 g

36. Mexican Beef Jerky

Preparation Time: 15 minutes

Cooking Time: 3 hours

Servings: 4

Ingredients:

- 11/2 pounds beef round, trimmed
- 1/2 cup Worcestershire sauce
- 1/2 cup low-sodium soy sauce
- 2 teaspoons honey
- 1 teaspoon liquid smoke
- 2 teaspoons onion powder
- 1/2 teaspoon red pepper flakes
- Ground black pepper, as required

Directions:

1. In a zip-top bag, place the beef and freeze for 1-2 hours to firm up.
2. Place the meat onto a cutting board and cut against the grain into 1/8-¼-inch strips.
3. In a large bowl, add the remaining ingredients and mix until well combined.
4. Add the steak slices and coat with the mixture generously.
5. Refrigerate to marinate for about 4-6 hours.
6. Remove the beef slices from bowl and with paper towels, pat dry them.

7. Divide the steak strips onto the cooking trays and arrange in an even layer.

8. Select "Dehydrate" and then adjust the temperature to 160 degrees F.

9. Set the timer for 3 hours and press the "Start".

10. When the display shows "Add Food" insert 1 tray in the top position and another in the center position.

11. After 11/2 hours, switch the position of cooking trays.

12. Meanwhile, in a small pan, add the remaining ingredients over medium heat and cook for about 10 minutes, stirring occasionally.

13. When cooking time is complete, remove the trays from Vortex.

Nutrition: Calories 372 Total Fat 10.7 g Saturated Fat 4 g Cholesterol 152 mg Sodium 2000 mg Total Carbs 12 g Fiber 0.2 g Sugar 11.3 g Protein 53.8 g

37. La Sweet & Spicy Meatballs

Preparation Time: 20 minutes

Cooking Time: 30 minutes

Servings: 8

Ingredients:

- For Meatballs:
- 2 pounds lean ground beef
- 2/3 cup quick-cooking oats
- 1/2 cup Ritz crackers, crushed
- 1 (5-ounce) can evaporated milk
- 2 large eggs, beaten lightly
- 1 teaspoon honey
- 1 tablespoon dried onion, minced
- 1 teaspoon garlic powder
- 1 teaspoon ground cumin
- Salt and ground black pepper, as required
- For Sauce:
- 1/3 cup orange marmalade
- 1/3 cup honey
- 1/3 cup brown sugar
- 2 tablespoons cornstarch
- 2 tablespoons soy sauce
- 1-2 tablespoons hot sauce
- 1 tablespoon Worcestershire sauce

Directions:

1. For meatballs: in a large bowl, add all the ingredients and mix until well combined.
2. Make 11/2-inch balls from the mixture.
3. Arrange half of the meatballs onto a cooking tray in a single layer.
4. Arrange the drip pan in the bottom of Instant Vortex plus Air Fryer Oven cooking chamber.
5. Select "Air Fry" and then adjust the temperature to 380 degrees F.
6. Set the timer for 15 minutes and press the "Start".
7. When the display shows "Add Food" insert the cooking tray in the center position.
8. When the display shows "Turn Food" turn the meatballs.
9. When cooking time is complete, remove the tray from Vortex.
10. Repeat with the remaining meatballs.
11. Meanwhile, for sauce: in a small pan, add all the ingredients over medium heat and cook until thickened, stirring continuously.
12. Serve the meatballs with the topping of sauce.

Nutrition: Calories 411 Total Fat 11.1 g Saturated Fat 4.1 g Cholesterol 153 mg Sodium 448 mg Total Carbs 38.8 g Fiber 1 g Sugar 28.1 g Protein 38.9 g

38. Spiced Seasoned Pork Shoulder

Preparation Time: 15 minutes

Cooking Time: 55 minutes

Servings: 6

Ingredients:

- 1 teaspoon ground cumin
- 1 teaspoon cayenne pepper
- 1 teaspoon garlic powder
- Salt and ground black pepper, as required
- 2 pounds skin-on pork shoulder

Directions:

1. In a small bowl, mix together the spices, salt and black pepper.
2. Arrange the pork shoulder onto a cutting board, skin-side down.
3. Season the inner side of pork shoulder with salt and black pepper.
4. With kitchen twines, tie the pork shoulder into a long round cylinder shape.
5. Season the outer side of pork shoulder with spice mixture.
6. Insert the rotisserie rod through the pork shoulder.
7. Insert the rotisserie forks, one on each side of the rod to secure the pork shoulder.
8. Arrange the drip pan in the bottom of Instant Vortex plus Air Fryer Oven cooking chamber.

9. Select "Roast" and then adjust the temperature to 350 degrees F.

10. Set the timer for 55 minutes and press the "Start".

11. When the display shows "Add Food" press the red lever down and load the left side of the rod into the Vortex.

12. Now, slide the rod's left side into the groove along the metal bar so it doesn't move.

13. Then, close the door and touch "Rotate".

14. When cooking time is complete, press the red lever to release the rod.

15. Remove the pork from Vortex and place onto a platter for about 10 minutes before slicing.

16. With a sharp knife, cut the pork shoulder into desired sized slices and serve.

Nutrition: Calories 445 Total Fat 32.5 g Saturated Fat 11.9 g Cholesterol 136 mg Sodium 131 mg Total Carbs 0.7 g Fiber 0.2 g Sugar 0.2 g Protein 35.4 g

39. Mexican Seasoned Pork Tenderloin

Preparation Time: 10 minutes

Cooking Time: 45 minutes

Servings: 5

Ingredients:

- 11/2 pounds pork tenderloin
- 2-3 tablespoons BBQ pork seasoning

Directions:

1. Rub the pork with seasoning generously.
2. Insert the rotisserie rod through the pork tenderloin.
3. Insert the rotisserie forks, one on each side of the rod to secure the pork tenderloin.
4. Arrange the drip pan in the bottom of Instant Vortex plus Air Fryer Oven cooking chamber.
5. Select "Roast" and then adjust the temperature to 360 degrees F.
6. Set the timer for 45 minutes and press the "Start".
7. When the display shows "Add Food" press the red lever down and load the left side of the rod into the Vortex.
8. Now, slide the rod's left side into the groove along the metal bar so it doesn't move.
9. Then, close the door and touch "Rotate".
10. When cooking time is complete, press the red lever to release the rod.

11. Remove the pork from Vortex and place onto a platter for about 10 minutes before slicing.
12. With a sharp knife, cut the roast into desired sized slices and serve.

Nutrition: Calories 195 Cholesterol 99 mg Sodium 116 mg Protein 35.6 g

40. Air Fryer Garlic Pork Tenderloin

Preparation Time: 15 minutes

Cooking Time: 20 minutes

Servings: 5

Ingredients:

- 11/2 pounds pork tenderloin
- Nonstick cooking spray
- 2 small heads roasted garlic
- Salt and ground black pepper, as required

Directions:

1. Lightly, spray all the sides of pork with cooking spray and then, season with salt and black pepper.
2. Now, rub the pork with roasted garlic.
3. Arrange the roast onto the lightly greased cooking tray.
4. Arrange the drip pan in the bottom of Instant Vortex plus Air Fryer Oven cooking chamber.
5. Select "Air Fry" and then adjust the temperature to 400 degrees F.
6. Set the timer for 20 minutes and press the "Start".
7. When the display shows "Add Food" insert the cooking tray in the center position.
8. When the display shows "Turn Food" turn the pork.
9. When cooking time is complete, remove the tray from Vortex and place the roast onto a platter for about 10 minutes before slicing.
10. With a sharp knife, cut the roast into desired sized slices and serve.

Nutrition: Calories 202 Total Fat 4.8 g Saturated Fat 1.6 g Cholesterol 99 mg Sodium 109 mg Total Carbs 1.7 g Fiber 0.1 g Sugar 0.1 g Protein 35.9 g

41. Sweetened Pork Tenderloin

Preparation Time: 15 minutes

Cooking Time: 20 minutes

Servings: 3

Ingredients:

- 1-pound pork tenderloin
- 2 tablespoons Sriracha
- 2 tablespoons honey
- Salt, as required

Directions:

1. Insert the rotisserie rod through the pork tenderloin.
2. Insert the rotisserie forks, one on each side of the rod to secure the pork tenderloin.
3. In a small bowl, add the Sriracha, honey and salt and mix well.
4. Brush the pork tenderloin with honey mixture evenly.
5. Arrange the drip pan in the bottom of Instant Vortex plus Air Fryer Oven cooking chamber.
6. Select "Air Fry" and then adjust the temperature to 350 degrees F.
7. Set the timer for 20 minutes and press the "Start".
8. When the display shows "Add Food" press the red lever down and load the left side of the rod into the Vortex.
9. Now, slide the rod's left side into the groove along the metal bar so it doesn't move.
10. Then, close the door and touch "Rotate".

11. When cooking time is complete, press the red lever to release the rod.

12. Remove the pork from Vortex and place onto a platter for about 10 minutes before slicing.

13. With a sharp knife, cut the roast into desired sized slices and serve.

Nutrition: Calories 269 Total Fat 5.3 g Saturated Fat 1.8 g Cholesterol 110 mg Sodium 207 mg Total Carbs 13.5 g Sugar 11.6 g Protein 39.7 g

DESSERTS RECIPES

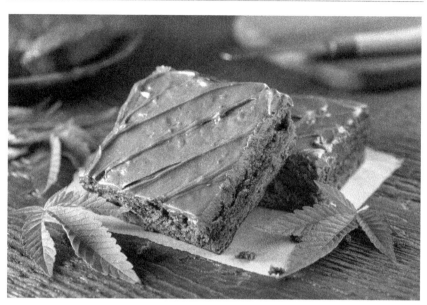

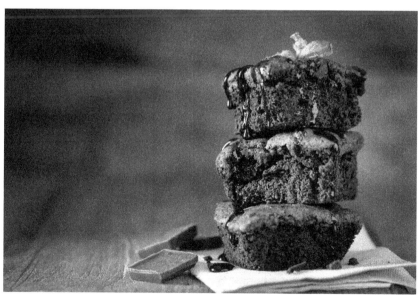

42. Beignets

Preparation Time: 20 minutes

Cooking Time: 6 minutes

Servings: 24

Ingredients:

- c. coconut milk
- 1/2 t. yeast
- tbsp. powdered sugar
- tbsp. melted coconut oil
- tbsp. aquafaba, from chickpeas
- t. vanilla
- c. flour

Directions:

1. Begin by mixing coconut milk, powdered sugar, and yeast in a small bowl.

2. Next start heating the coconut milk until it is warm to the touch but not hot. Then add to your mixture from the small bowl and let sit 10 minutes to allow the yeast to foam.

3. Next using the paddle attachment on a stand mixer add the vanilla, aquafaba, coconut oil, and mix. Then add flour one cup at a time.

4. As flour is missing the dough should begin to come away from the sides, if you have a dough hook switch from paddle to the dough hook.

5. Allow dough to knead in the mixer for about 3 minutes dough will be wet, but you should be able to scrape it out and form into balls with your hands.

6. Place the dough in mixing bowl and cover with a clean towel and allow to rise for 1 hour.

7. On a large clean cutting board sprinkle some flour and pat out the dough into a rectangle shape about 1/3-inch thick. Then Cut into 24 squares and allow to proof for 30 minutes.

8. Cooking in batches add 3 to 6 beignets at a time cook at 390 for 3 minutes then turn and allow to fry 3 more minutes or until golden brown.

9. Sprinkle with powdered sugar and enjoy.

Nutrition: Calories: 102 Net Carbs: 15 g Fat: 3 g Protein: 3 g

43. S'more

Preparation Time: 10 minutes

Cooking Time: 6 minutes

Servings: 8

Ingredients:

- 4 marshmallows
- Heresy bar
- 8 graham cracker squares

Directions:

1. Begin by placing a marshmallow on a graham cracker
2. Place in the air fryer and roast marshmallow at 400 for 6 minutes
3. Remove from air fryer and top with chocolate and graham cracker square and enjoy

Nutrition: Calories: 225 Net Carbs: 38 g Fat: 7 g Protein: 2 g

44. Fried Oreos

Preparation Time: 10 minutes

Cooking Time: 5 minutes

Servings: 9

Ingredients:

- 9 Oreo cookies
- Crescent roll sheet

Directions:

1. Begin by opening crescent roll and spreading it on a work surface then cut 9 even squares.

2. Place one Oreo into each square and wrap dough around the cookie.

3. Lightly spray the outside of the wrapped cookies with cooking spray and place in the fryer and fry at 360 for 2 minutes, then flip and fry an additional 2 minutes.

4. Sprinkle tops of Oreos with powdered sugar and enjoy.

Nutrition: Calories: 58 Net Carbs: 8.4 g Fat: 2.6 g Protein: 0.6 g

45. Fig Egg Rolls

Preparation Time: 15 minutes

Cooking Time: 5 minutes

Servings: 15

Ingredients:

- ¼ c. sugar
- 2 tbsp. butter, melted
- 15 egg roll wrappers
- oz. jar fig jam
- 16 oz. cream cheese
- 1/2 c. sugar
- tsp. Cinnamon
- tsp. Lemon Juice
- 1 tsp. Vanilla extract

Directions:

1. Begin by adding lemon juice, sugar, cream cheese, and vanilla extract into a mixer and whipping about 2 minutes to combine.
2. Remove the mixture and place into a pastry bag
3. Next stir the jam in the jar so it is loosened and easy to be scooped with a spoon.
4. Next layout the egg roll wrappers in a diamond shape with the point facing you.

5. In the center of the egg roll pipe approximately 2 tablespoons of cream cheese mixture then top with a tablespoon of jam.
6. Using a pastry brush to coat the edges of the egg roll wrapper with water.
7. Fold the bottom over the filling and secure tightly, then fold each side in and roll the egg roll up the rest of the way.
8. Next spray both sides with cooking spray.
9. Then allow the egg rolls to rest at room temperature
10. Next place 4-5 egg rolls in air fryer basket and fry at 370 for 5 minutes or until egg rolls are golden brown.
11. Remove egg rolls and allow to cool
12. After all egg rolls are cooked brush the tops with melted butter and sprinkle with cinnamon and sugar.
13. Serve at room temperature.

Nutrition: Calories: 297 Net Carbs: 41.5 g Fat: 12.6 g Protein: 5.5 g

46. Grilled Pineapple

Preparation Time: 10 minutes

Cooking Time: 10 minutes

Servings: 4

Ingredients:

- 3 tbsp. melted butter
- 2 t. cinnamon, ground
- 1/2 c. brown sugar
- pineapple, peeled – cored and cut into spears

Directions:

1. Begin by using a small bowl to mix together cinnamon and brown sugar.
2. Next brush pineapple with melted butter to coat all sides then toss in cinnamon sugar until spears are well coated.
3. Spray air fryer with cooking spray and add pineapple fry at 400 for 5 minutes.
4. Brush with additional butter and fry another 5 minutes or until sugar is bubbling.

Nutrition: Calories: 295 Net Carbs: 57 g Fat: 8 g Protein: 1 g

47. Chocolate Covered Strawberry S'more

Preparation Time: 10 minutes

Cooking Time: 6 minutes

Servings: 8

Ingredients:

- 4 marshmallows
- 4 t. Nutella
- 8 strawberries sliced
- 8 chocolate graham cracker squares

Directions:

1. Begin by placing a marshmallow on the chocolate graham cracker
2. Place in the basket of air fryer and roast marshmallow for 6 minutes with a temperature of 400
3. Remove from air fryer, and top with 2 slices of strawberry and Nutella then add top graham cracker square and enjoy.

Nutrition: Calories: 225 Net Carbs: 38 g Protein: 2 g Fat: 7 g

48. Air Fryer Oven Peppermint Lava Cake

Preparation Time: 15 minutes

Cooking Time: 15 minutes

Servings: 4

Ingredients:

- 2 large eggs
- 2/3 cups semisweet chocolate chips
- 1 tsp. peppermint extract
- 1/2 cup cubed butter
- 6 tablespoons all- purpose flour
- 2large egg yolks
- 2 tablespoons crushed peppermint candies (optional)
- 1 cup confectioners' sugar

Directions:

1. Preheat air fryer oven to 375F

2. Melt butter and chocolate chips in microwave safe bowl for 30 seconds and stir until smooth. Whisk in eggs, egg yolks, confectioners' sugars and extract until blended. Fold in flout

3. Grease and flour ramekins, pour batter into ramekins but avoid overfilling it

4. Place ramekins in air fryer oven basket and cook for 10 to 15 minutes until thermometer reads 160F

5. Remove and allow it sit for 5 minutes, sprinkle with crush candies and enjoy.

Nutrition: Calories 367 Total Fat 19.2 g Saturated Fat 9.5 g Cholesterol 124 mg Sodium 265 mg Total Carbs 53.6 g Fiber 2.7 g Sugar 37.8 g Protein 6.4 g

49. Air Fryer Oven Chocolate Cake

Preparation Time: 15 minutes

Cooking Time: 20 minutes

Servings: 4

Ingredients:

- 3 eggs
- 1/2 cup sour cream
- 1 cup flour
- 2/3 cup sugar
- 1 stick butter room temperature
- 1/3 cup cocoa powder
- 1 teaspoon baking powder
- 1/2 teaspoon baking soda
- 2 teaspoons vanilla

Directions:

1. Preheat Air fryer oven to 320 degrees
2. Mix ingredients on low heat and pour into oven attachment
3. Place in Air fryer oven basket and Set timer to 25 minutes
4. Once timer rings, insert use toothpick to see if cake is done.
5. Cool cake on a wire rack
6. Ice with your favorite chocolate frosting

Nutrition: Calories 300 Total Fat 12 g Saturated 7.4 g Cholesterol 31 mg Sodium 122 mg Total Carbs 46.7 g Fiber 2.3 g Sugar 23.3g Protein 3.3 g

50. Air Fryer Oven Zucchini Fritters

Preparation Time: 15 minutes

Cooking Time: 15 minutes

Servings: 8

Ingredients:

- 100 g Plain Flour
- 1 Medium Egg beaten
- 5 Tbsp Milk
- 150 g Grated Courgette
- 75 g Spring Onion thinly sliced
- 25 g Cheddar Cheese grated
- 1 Tbsp Mixed Herbs
- Salt & Pepper

Directions:

1. Preheat the air fryer oven to 360F.

2. Grate the zucchini making sure to remove excess moisture.

3. Put plain flour into a bowl and add the seasoning. Whisk the egg and milk and then add to the flour to make a smooth batter. Stir in the cheese, add in the zucchini and the spring onion and mix well.

4. Make them into small burger shapes and place in the Air fryer oven.

5. Cook on a 360f temperature for 6 minutes or until fully cooked.

6. Serve with dollop of mayonnaise

Nutrition: Calories 191 Total Fat 16.5 g Saturated Fat 3 g Cholesterol 47 mg Sodium 54 mg Total Carbs 14.8 g Fiber 3.2 g Sugar 9.7 g Protein 6.8 g

CPSIA information can be obtained
at www.ICGtesting.com
Printed in the USA
BVHW041000120321
602396BV00016B/316